REINVENT AGING

The Over 50 Fitness Guide to Improve
Energy, Strength, and Balance

REINVENT AGING

The Over 50 Fitness Guide to Improve
Energy, Strength, and Balance

Aubrey Reinmiller

Published by Niche Pressworks

Before beginning any exercise program, check with your doctor for clearance.

Publishing, composition, and design managed by Niche Pressworks

http://nichepressworks.com

ISBN Print: 978-1-946533-04-3

ISBN Digital: 978-1-946533-05-0

Dedication

I dedicate this book in loving memory of my grandparents: Poppop, Mommom, and Granddad, with whom I wish I had many more days; and to my parents, who I hope have many healthy, active years with their grandkids ahead of them.

Thank you to my husband, Andrew, for always being there for me and for being a great hands-on dad.

Table of Contents

Dan Ritchie, PhD
Foreword

Will you have the ability and energy to travel halfway across the globe on an amazing adventure when you are pushing seventy? Would you like to?

Bev first came to us in her early sixties when she was healthy, but not fit. She needed to lose weight and get much stronger. A few years later, her health changed dramatically after a bad case of the flu. She spent several months in special medical treatments after she contracted a rare autoimmune disease that attacked her muscles. When she came back to us in her mid-sixties, she was weak and not physically ready for her bucket list trip to Antarctica. The funny thing was her biggest goal was to be able to jump out of a zodiac boat—so "no young kid will grab me by the butt and toss me out." We began her training with many basic functional strength movements, eventually progressing to power and jumping movements to move her entire body quickly. Keep in mind that while she claimed to be five feet tall, she was more like four feet ten, so the rubber zodiac boats came up to her waist, and she had to be able to jump out as they beached. This was not going to be a two-to-three-month training program. It took six months to recover what she had lost from her illness. Then we began the training to make sure she could move quickly and powerfully, so she could hop in and out of those boats like she was thirty-five not sixty-five.

Had she been unprepared, that trip to Antarctica may not have been the lifetime experience with her husband as it was. The over one thousand pictures they brought back and shared with us told the real story; it was a trip they would never forget. And Bev was proud to report she had no trouble hopping in and out of the Zodiac boats as they beached. "No young guy had to grab me by the rear and hoist me overboard!"

Many people can afford to go on adventures, but no longer have the ability to really enjoy them. It highlights a very important fact—age should *never* be a reason for slowing down and giving in. Too many great adventures are still to come in life.

Over the years, we have seen thousands of middle-aged and older adults improve the quality of their life through transformational exercise programs that maximize physical function. This is why it is so important that you have this book in your hand right now—at this very moment in time. This is why we founded the Functional Aging Institute with the ultimate goal of improving the lives of people just like you all around the globe!

Our goal is to help people realize that they can keep doing all the things they need to do, like to do, and want to do for a very long time—as long as they follow the exercise principles and strategies outlined in this book.

Whether it is taking the grandchildren to Disney, taking on a new career, climbing mountains, extending the years you get to play golf and tennis, or traveling around the world—you can do it all into your seventies, eighties, and nineties with greater ease and less pain.

This is where the Functional Aging Training model and the Functional Aging Institute comes in. We are now in sixteen countries, forty-six of fifty states in the United States and growing. We are on our way to our goal of having ten thousand certified Functional Aging Specialists around the world who will guide ten to twenty million people toward a different aging trajectory; one that allows people like you to look forward to their next twenty to thirty years with joyful anticipation, knowing you are doing the best you can to stay healthy and functional. By choosing to connect yourself with Aubrey Reinmiller and Vitality Fitness, you are making a decision that will enrich your life, and the lives of all the people you love, for generations to come. We are grateful to contribute to that vision.

Dan Ritchie, PhD

Co-founder, Functional Aging Institute

Preface

Imagine it is Thanksgiving Day. You sit down at the table, joining extended family while scrumptious aromas fill the air. You join your family to give thanks and then suddenly you hear someone shouting, "She's choking! Do the Heimlich maneuver!" Everyone stands up and your cousin rushes to your great-aunt and performs the Heimlich maneuver. A piece of roll flies across the table! While everyone had bowed their heads, our ninety-five-year-old aunt had taken the opportunity to swallow an entire dinner roll despite medical conditions forbidding her to eat solids. This happened one year at my family Thanksgiving dinner. Never a dull moment!

My love of older folks developed early as I grew up close to my grandparents, great-aunts and -uncles. Many of these relatives were able to move into the same senior living apartment building. Much of my childhood was spent going from floor to floor having a different adventure with each of them. I learned card games, ate a lot of candy, and enjoyed listening to stories.

As my relatives aged, I saw how difficult it became for them to get around. Many of them had physical therapy to help them to manage their aches and pains and to stay active. It was seeing how this important service helped my loved ones that led me to decide early on that I would pursue a career in physical therapy.

During my first job in physical therapy, I worked with young athletes. I thought it would be fun to help them resume their sport after injury. While working with the athletes had its interesting moments, I found the most joy working with older adults. Older adults knew the benefits of hard work. They would more willingly comply with my exercise requests and in turn saw life-changing results. Of course, we would joke about their "favorite" exercises being the ones they dreaded the most. I found this to be the most rewarding work.

After many years in physical therapy, I was convinced there was a need for expert guidance once physical therapy had ended. With the limitations on insurance coverage increasing each year, many patients were discharged before they fully recovered, especially when it came to those with more complex medical conditions. Frequently, patients would tell me they tried to work with a personal trainer in a big box gym and had been pushed too hard, too fast, and found themselves frustrated and further injured.

Vitality Fitness and Wellness was founded as a solution to the problem and a way in which I could provide expert personal training services to those who needed more guidance after their physical therapy benefits had run out. Vitality Fitness and Wellness has evolved to serve those that are recovering from injury or dealing with a chronic medical condition and to serve healthy boomers and seniors who want to remain active.

The boomer generation is different than their parents. They have become the sandwich generation, caring for their aging parents at the same time they are caring for their children. The boomer generation is also the first generation to make fitness fun and incorporate it into a lifestyle. As such, they see the importance of remaining active and independent for as long as possible. For this to occur, exercise is vital. Often, with the demands of life, exercise takes a back seat. I encourage you to get back into it. It is not too late.

Vitality Fitness and Wellness provides one-on-one and small group personal training for older adults to improve strength, balance, endurance, posture, and flexibility to help you feel better and move better. We use a functional fitness approach where exercises are performed in all three planes of motion to mimic the motions of daily life. I wrote this book as a guide for those over fifty who would like to start or resume fitness training so they can enjoy their life for many years to come. Let us reinvent aging together!

Chapter 1
Start Now

"Get up offa that thing..."
—James Brown

Exercise. To many people that sounds like a dirty word. Excuses abound. We know it is important but we put it off. Maybe it has been years since you have exercised; maybe an injury or health condition has put exercise on hold; maybe you find the gym or the latest exercise trend intimidating. What your body needs at age fifty, sixty, and beyond is different from what a twenty-year-old needs. The difficulty of not knowing where to start can be paralyzing to your aspirations of a healthy lifestyle. In the chapters of this book, let us put your mind at ease and walk you through the right exercises for your body.

The boomer generation has seen how their parents and grandparents have aged and they want something different. Boomers today are more active than any previous generation. They are not strangers to fitness as the fitness revolution was born when baby boomers were young. The Presidential Physical Fitness Award program began in 1966 with a movement to encourage youth to be more active. Exercise became fun with the birth of such fitness options as dance aerobics, running, health clubs, and sports clubs. However, like many fads somewhere along the way, exercise dwindled. Whether it is a result of the busy schedules of the middle-aged with kids, aging parents, and careers or the distractions of technology, we have gone astray from the fun of exercise and it has become the last task on our to do list and never gets done.

The age-in-place movement is another way of life that developed mainly from the baby boomers. It began with a desire to live at home for as long as possible and to stay out of nursing homes. From there, age-in-place villages have been established in different areas of the country to support this practice. In the DC metro area alone, we already have at least twenty villages. In order to remain at home, our bodies must stay strong to be able to climb the stairs, put away the groceries, and keep active for these and other everyday activities. Exercise may not excite you, but we want you to be excited that with exercise you can move with more ease, have better strength, balance, and endurance to enjoy an active lifestyle.

Take, for example, our client Linda who recently retired after working in the school system. Linda's mother passed away a few years ago after an extended period of ill health. Linda put her own needs on hold while caring for her mother. She used to be very active and was frustrated with how tight and sore she had become. She never thought this would happen to her.

Linda enjoyed travel, another aspect of her life that was put on hold while caring for her mother. She planned a trip to Israel with her husband. She was excited for the trip, but knew it would include long days with a lot of walking, uneven ground, and many sets of stairs. She was not sure she could keep up. She also struggled with back pain that flared up every now and then and worried it would occur during her trip. For Linda to enjoy her trip to the fullest, we chose exercises to improve the strength in her legs for stair climbing, her balance for maneuvering on uneven terrain while taking in the sights around her, her core strength to prevent back pain, and her overall endurance to travel long days. Linda did not realize she could feel so good at her age. Not only did she fully enjoy her trip, everyday tasks were much easier when she got home.

As you age, exercise becomes vital to maintaining a strong body in order to enjoy all the activities you are passionate about. We are ready to steer you on the right track and help you discover that fitness does not have to be intimidating. We want you to stay healthy for yourself, your family, your job, your hobbies, and your life!

The three most important areas to focus on with exercise as we age are posture, balance, and strength. In the following chapters, I will explain more about each of these aspects and give examples of exercises to address these aspects.

Chapter 2
Posture

"A good stance and posture reflect a good state of mind."
—MORIHEI UESHIBA

Look and Feel Your Best

Good posture is essential to a good appearance. More importantly, it is essential to overall wellness. Poor posture can cause aches and pains or even numbness in the limbs. Bad habits developed in childhood generate these warning signs, which may start as early as the twenties. Other consequences include falls, fractures, and spinal compression. Muscle imbalances can lead to pain and lack of function. Related conditions arise in later years: "sitting disease," osteoporosis, and arthritis. You can prevent these conditions with proper exercise and attention to your posture.

Do you want to keep doing the activities you enjoy? The guidance of an experienced personal trainer will help you choose the right exercises, correct your posture, and increase your flexibility.

Sitting Disease

Does your job involve a lot of computer work? How long is your commute? The DC metro area is one of the worst areas for traffic. Just getting out to the grocery store can be an all-day event. How many hours a day do you spend sitting? If you use an activity tracker, how often do you reach the recommended ten thousand steps a day? Many of us underestimate the amount of time we spend sitting each day. Sitting too long can affect our body's alignment and cause painful conditions to arise.

Without correct posture, pressure on the discs reduces the space between vertebrae. Over time, the chest muscles shorten and the upper back muscles weaken. Shoulder muscles, not the body's powerhouse muscles, take over the task of holding up the head. The wrong muscles working overtime become muscle imbalances, leading to pain, dysfunction, and pressure on the nerves and spine. Strengthen the upper back and postural muscles and stretch the chest and neck muscles so they can support an improved seated position. At the end of this chapter, you will see some good examples of exercises to get you started.

Inactivity affects posture, and along with it, overall health. More and more studies link sedentary behavior to poor health. "Sitting disease" is the term that links a sedentary lifestyle to health issues such as diabetes, cognitive decline, certain cancers, and cardiovascular disease. A study done by the Mayo Clinic revealed that 50 to 70 percent of people spend six or more hours sitting every day. In addition, 20 to 35 percent of people spend four hours or more watching TV each day. (Average American watches five hours of TV per day, report shows, David Hinckley, 3/5/14).

"Today, our bodies are breaking down from obesity, high blood pressure, diabetes, cancer, depression, and the cascade of health ills and everyday malaise that come from what scientists have named sitting disease."
—James Levine, MD, PhD (What are the risks of sitting too much?, mayoclinic.org)

For many years, Jack worked long hours seated at his desk. His commute added hours to his physically inactive workday. At long last, Jack happily joined his wife in retirement, anticipating the fulfillment of his dream for their "Golden Years."

Almost immediately, the dream faded as neck pain kept him off the golf course. Soon, the pain began to radiate down his arm. One day, he reached down to pick up a piece of paper and the pain worsened. Jack was baffled. How could such a simple act aggravate his body? That was the straw that broke the camel's back. Jack had a herniated disc in his neck.

Jack was not much for exercise, except for his golf game, so he was hesitant to start exercising at his age. He worried that starting now would only cause more injury. His doctor suggested surgery to relieve the compression in his spine, but Jack was reluctant to go under the knife. Years hunched over his desk had left Jack with a rounded upper back and forward head posture. Jack had imagined spending his hard-earned retirement playing golf and traveling to sunny beaches. Instead, he was plagued with pain and fatigue.

He looked for alternative treatments and found Vitality Fitness & Wellness. Jack made the decision to turn his life around by starting a regular exercise routine. At first, we worked together a few times a week on exercises to strengthen his upper back. Next, we worked on exercises to stretch his neck and chest to allow his posture to improve. Before long, Jack's pain had decreased and the numbness in his arm was gone. Jack was able to avoid surgery and get back to playing golf, his favorite activity. Even his doctor was surprised at the gains that Jack had made from a few months of the right exercises!

Tips to correct your posture at a desk:

- Have someone take a picture of you when you are at your desk and unaware of being photographed.

- Post that picture as a reminder to adjust your posture while you are working.

- Every time you finish a task, look away from your screen, sit up tall, and take three deep breaths. Roll your shoulders back, adjust to your best posture, and get back to work.

- Scoot your bottom all the way back into your chair so that your back can use the support of the chair.

- Keep your feet flat—adjust the chair or grab a small box to rest your feet on.

- Directly face the task you are working on.

- Every two hours be sure to stand up and stretch or take a quick walk.

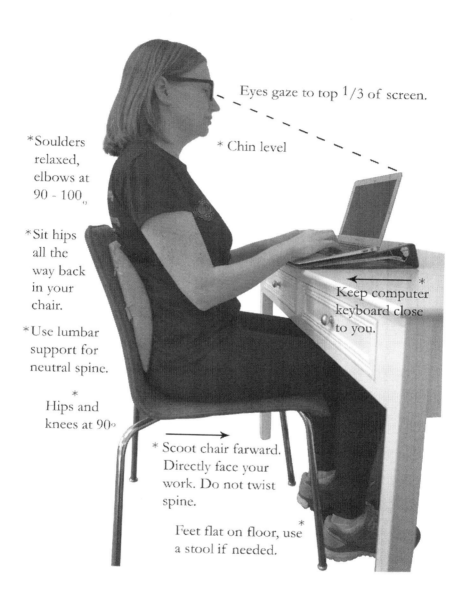

Eyes gaze to top 1/3 of screen.

*Soulders
relaxed,
elbows at
90 - 100₀

* Chin level

*Sit hips
all the
way back
in your
chair.

*Use lumbar
support for
neutral spine.

*
Keep computer
keyboard close
to you.

*
Hips and
knees at 90°

* Scoot chair farward.
Directly face your
work. Do not twist
spine.

Feet flat on floor, use *
a stool if needed.

Osteoporosis

Another condition affecting posture is Osteoporosis. Osteoporosis is a disease in which your bones lose density. They become porous and more prone to fractures. This most commonly occurs in the spine, wrist, hip, and shoulder. Osteoporosis is most common in women because estrogen levels drop after menopause causing bone loss. Most women are concerned about their posture as they age. They want to avoid the rounded upper back they have seen in their mothers and grandmothers. This rounded posture is an excessive kyphosis, or dowager's hump, caused by the thinning of the vertebrae from bone loss related to osteoporosis. Excessive kyphosis is not only unsightly—it can lead to pain, trouble breathing, and lack of range of motion in the neck, back, and shoulders.

Practicing good posture can also reduce your risk of falls by keeping your center of gravity in line. Falls are much more detrimental when you have osteoporosis due to the increased risk of bone fracture. In fact, the most common reason for broken bones among older adults is osteoporosis. According to the National Osteoporosis Foundation, half of all adults over fifty are at risk of breaking a bone and should be concerned about bone health. (National Osteoporosis Foundation, nof. org) One of the main ways to prevent osteoporosis and improve posture is through exercise, which increases bone strength. To increase bone strength, weight bearing and resistance exercises are the best type of exercise. Our programs incorporate body weight exercises to improve your posture and reduce the risk of osteoporosis. Here are a few examples:

Weight Bearing Exercises to Reduce Osteoporosis Risk and Improve Posture:

Wall pushup

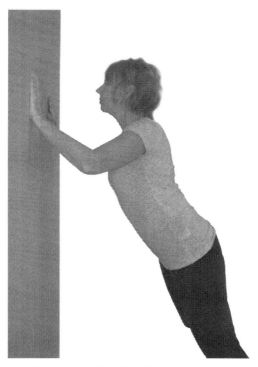

1. Step away from wall, further away increases the challenge.
2. Place hands on wall; keep body in straight line.
3. Bend elbows and lower slowly towards wall.
4. Push out without locking elbows.
5. Do 1-3 sets of 10 repetitions.

    **Note about exercise dose-age: In general strengthening exercises should be performed 3 times a week. Start with 1-2 sets of 10 and progress to 3 sets of 10 before progressing the exercise.

Bird dog

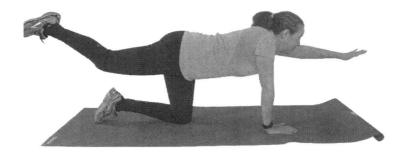

1. Start on hands and knees, shoulders directly over wrists, hips over knees.
2. Tuck in tummy muscles and gently squeeze shoulder blades.
3. Reach out opposite arm and leg. Keep hips level.
4. Hold 5 seconds. Do 10 times on each side. Work up to 3 sets.

Mountain climbers

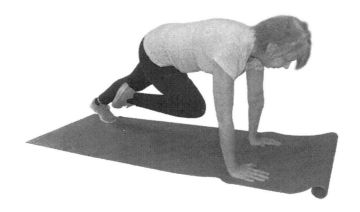

1. Get down on hands and knees. Shoulders should be directly over wrists.
2. Raise your knees from floor into plank position.
3. March knee towards opposite arm.
4. Do 5 times, alternating knees. Work up to 3 sets. (For less intensity, perform this against a sturdy chair seat or table with your body at an incline.)

Planks (modified and regular)

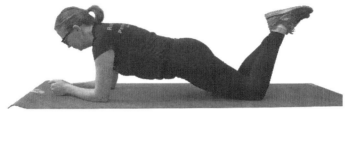

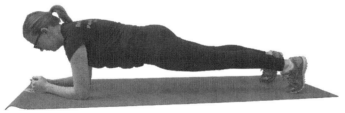

1. Place forearms on mat. Rise up on knees for modified plank or toes for plank.
2. Tuck stomach muscles in. Keep body in line, keep bottom down. Shoulders should be directly over elbows.
3. Hold for 5-10 seconds. Do 2-3 reps. Slowly increase the length of hold. If back pain, or losing form, stop and hold for less time.

Osteoarthritis

Most people assume joint pain is an inevitable part of getting older. Maybe you remember your mother referring to "old Arthur coming back to town" as she complained about more difficulty with climbing the stairs, bending down, or other daily activities. Osteoarthritis occurs when the cartilage, which is the protective covering at the end of bones, begins to wear away allowing bone to rub against bone. It occurs most commonly in the weight-bearing joints of the body: knees, hips, and back. Arthritis can cause symptoms such as achiness, pain, stiffness, swelling, and decreased range of motion. It may be exacerbated by carrying excess weight, family history, age, and poor alignment of our bodies. While we cannot control all of those risk factors, we can work on our posture and maintain a healthy weight.

Chronic poor posture can cause excess pressure on our joints increasing symptoms of arthritis. Performing the right exercises can improve the alignment of our bodies and decrease the pressure on our joints. It is possible to have arthritis without having any symptoms, although most times symptoms will manifest in time. Those with muscle imbalances will notice more pain and symptoms from arthritis. If you are proactive and start an appropriate exercise program to address these muscle imbalances, you can stay active and pain free.

When you are in pain and experiencing the symptoms of arthritis, exercise might be the last thing on your mind. However, it is an important part of healing. Synovial fluid is the thick liquid located in the joints that lubricates the joints during movement, much like how motor oil keeps the engine in your car from seizing up. Oftentimes when our body is in pain, the instinct is to protect the area by limiting motion. For example, if you are experiencing shoulder pain, it is tempting to keep your shoulder still and close to your body to protect it like a broken wing. However, this is the worst thing you can do for your body. As long as we know the limb is not broken and the pain is from arthritis, it is important to keep the shoulder moving through small motion to allow the synovial fluid to bathe the joint to ease motion and reduce pain. Good posture takes constant attention and hard work. It is important to pay attention to your posture and correct it often. Here are a few tips to keep in mind when you are standing for longer periods.

Tips for standing with good posture:

- Do not lock your knees.
- Try to stand with even weight on each leg; do not sit into one hip.
- Keep your upper body lifted as if someone is pulling a string from the top of your head.
- Keep your chest open and your shoulders relaxed down and back. (Think about it right now. Are your shoulders truly relaxed?)
- Keep your abdominal muscles tucked in with your pelvis level and not tipped forward.
- Remember to choose good, supportive footwear. Posture starts from the feet up.

Mary Anne was a high school English teacher with two young grandchildren. She was very active with her community, her job, and her family. Her exercise routine was her regular walking group with some coworkers. Being a teacher and on her feet most of the day, she often reached her goal of ten thousand daily steps with her fitness tracker. Even though she regularly exercised, she noticed she was having some trouble getting up and down from the floor when her grandson asked her to play trains, his favorite game. Mary Anne also began to develop some shoulder pain. She had trouble with driving, reaching for her seatbelt, and picking up her grandkids. She experienced an overall achiness. Her doctor said she had some arthritis. Mary Anne ignored the problem for a while, as many of us do, hoping it would resolve itself. Her pain did not go away and she developed a frozen shoulder, adhesive capsulitis.

Mary Anne went to physical therapy for her shoulder, but also decided she might need exercise advice. She joined our group training and supplemented her physical therapy with exercises for posture and strength as guided by our personal trainers. She realized her walking group challenged her aerobically, but did not challenge her strength. With guidance for safe, effective stretching and strengthening of her postural, she was able to get rid of her shoulder pain. Mary Anne also noticed a difference in her energy levels and was able to do the hills in her walking group faster than her coworkers were. Most importantly, she was able to get up and down to play trains with her grandson.

Sample Exercises:

Row

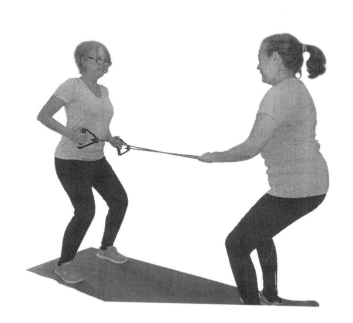

1. Can anchor band with doorway anchor or perform with a partner. Cross your bands and you can both perform!
2. Stand feet shoulder-width apart; gently bend your knees.
3. Keep elbows close to your body and hands with thumb up position.
4. Pull your elbows back and squeeze your shoulder blades together. Do not hunch your shoulders. Keep your stomach muscles tight. Do not arch your back.
5. Do 1-3 sets of 10 repetitions.

Warrior cheerleader

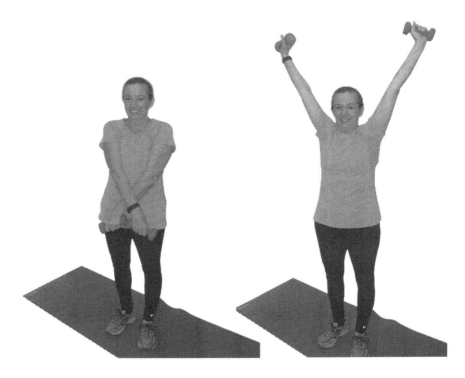

1. Stand feet shoulder-width apart. Holding light weights (1-3#).
2. Cross arms in front of you for warrior pose.
3. Uncross arms creating a "V" with your arms for cheerleader pose. Do not hunch your shoulders and squeeze your shoulder blades. Keep stomach muscles in tight; do not lean back.
4. Do 1-3 sets of 10.

Deadlift

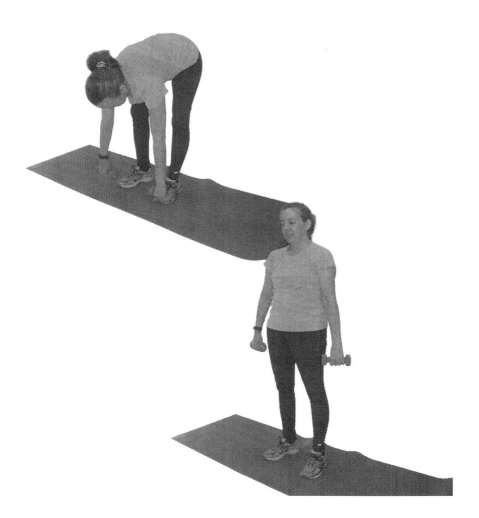

1. Hold light weights by your side.
2. Keep back straight and slowly lower down.
3. Squeeze your glutes, raise up, keeping your back straight, arms by your side.
4. Do 1-3 sets of 10 reps.

Doorway stretch

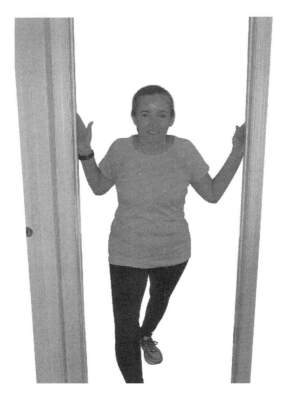

1. Place hands on doorway, relax shoulders, and bring elbows down.
2. Take a step forward and keep back straight.
3. Gently lean in until you feel a stretch in the front of your chest.
4. Hold for 30 seconds. Repeat 2-3 times.

**Note about stretching dose-age: Stretches can be performed daily with 30 second hold. Perform each stretch 1-3 times. Keep breathing! If you notice you hold your breath, focus on holding for 4-5 deep breaths instead of seconds.

UT stretch

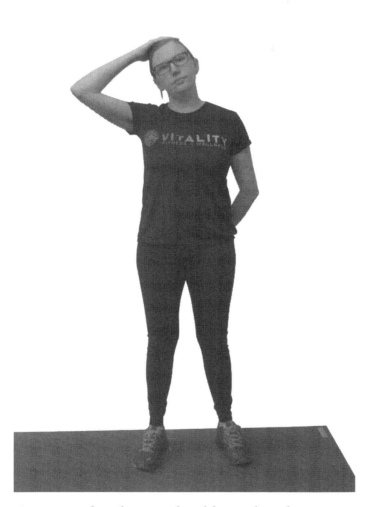

1. Sit or stand with your shoulders relaxed.
2. Gently tilt your head to the side, keep looking forward.
3. Gently use other hand to apply pressure if necessary.
4. Hold 30 seconds. Do 1-3 repetitions.

Hamstring stretch

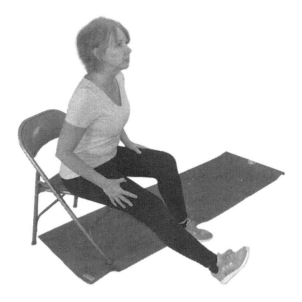

1. Sit at the front edge of a sturdy chair.
2. Place one leg straight out in front of you with the heel down and toes upwards.
3. Keep your back straight, gently lean forward until you feel a stretch behind your thigh.
4. Hold for 30 seconds. Do 1-3 times.

Chapter 3
Balance

"Fitness is a journey, not a destination; you must continue for the rest of your life."
—KENNETH COOPER

One of the biggest concerns of older adults today is balance. Are you worried about falling? Have you had a fall? Balance will decline as we age unless we continue to exercise to improve our balance and strength. Falls are the leading cause of injury among older adults, resulting in an older adult seeking treatment in the Emergency Room for an injury every fifteen seconds. (National Council on Aging, ncoa.org) Even the fear of falling can have a large impact on a person's quality of life by causing them to limit their activities. Falls are not an inevitable part of aging, and with a commitment to exercise, they can be prevented.

Balance has three components: our vision, our proprioception, and our vestibular system. All three of these systems decline as we get older, but with exercise, we can help to sharpen these systems and improve balance. A healthy visual system allows you to sense where your body is in relation to your surroundings. If you have difficulty seeing due to poor vision or dimly lit areas, you will have more trouble maintaining your balance and judging distance or obstacles.

Proprioception is a system made up of special sensors in your body's muscles, tendons, and joints that allow you to understand where your body is in space. This system, along with our body's reflexes, slows as we age, creating greater challenges to our balance. The final component, the vestibular system, is a set of three tubes in the inner ear lined with tiny hairs that send signals to the brain to tell our brains the position of our head. As we get older, we start to lose the small hairs that line these tubes making it much more difficult for the brain to receive the right signals. In this section, we will describe certain exercises you can do to help sharpen all three of these systems to promote better balance.

Safety tips:

- Have your vision checked regularly; at least every year.

- Be mindful of medications and their side effects.

- Have your doctor or pharmacist review your medications to check interactions and side effects.

- Keep pathways in your home clear and free of clutter. Remove papers, books, obstacles, clothes, and shoes, especially around stairs and thresholds.

- Remove throw rugs, as they are trip-hazards. If necessary, secure edges with non-slip pads or double-sided tape.

- Improve lighting in your home and along outdoor pathways.

- Wear supportive shoes. Avoid slippers that can fall off or become worn or damaged.

Simple Balance Test:

Is your balance in top shape or do you need to improve it? There are many balance tests out there but this is a simple test you can do at home with a partner. Be sure to be safe. If you are unsure of your abilities, try this test with someone steady spotting you.

1. Stand with your back to a corner or near a sturdy countertop.
2. Stand on one leg.
3. Time how long you can stand without touching with your hands or tapping your foot down.
4. Repeat three times and divide the total of seconds by three. Check your score against the norms below for your age group.
5. Try it again with your eyes closed.

Balance norms (in seconds):

Age	50-59	60-69	70-79	80-99
Male	EO:38 EC:8.6	EO:33.8 EC:5.1	EO:25.9 EC:2.6	EO:8.7 EC:1.8
Female	EO:36 EC:7.9	EO:30.4 EC:3.6	EO:16.7 EC:3.7	EO:10.6 EC:8.7

(Springer et al, 2007)   EO= Eyes Open, EC= Eyes Closed

Types of Balance:

There are two types of balance: static and dynamic. Our bodies need practice with both types to be safe and steady. Static balance is how steady you are when you are standing still. Examples from your daily life include brushing your teeth, cooking at the stove, and reaching into the closet or cabinet. Dynamic balance is when your body is in motion. Some examples of this type of balance from your daily life include picking up a bag of groceries, walking up and down the stairs, walking down the street while looking around, walking through a narrow passage, and bending down to pick up something from the floor. In our programs, our personal trainers incorporate both types of balance to challenge your body and provide you with the best possible workout routine. During static balance exercises, we can challenge your balance by changing the position of your feet from a wider base of support to a narrower base of support. Some examples of these stances include:

Rhomberg

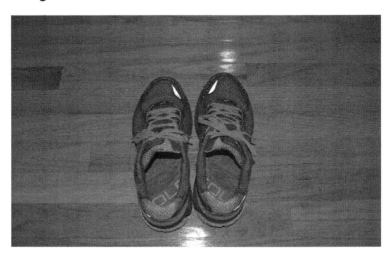

Half tandem

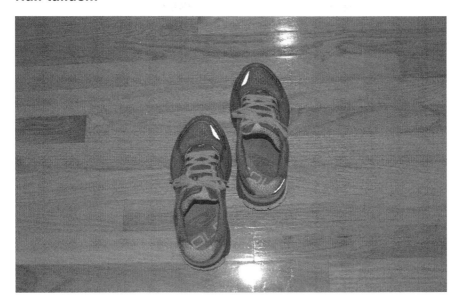

Tandem

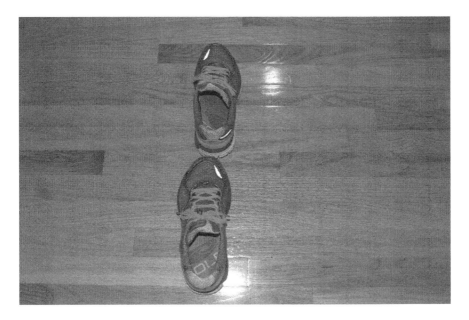

Partial single leg stance

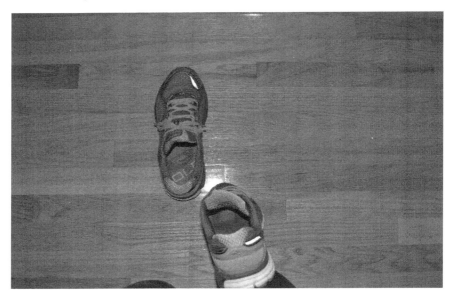

Single leg stance

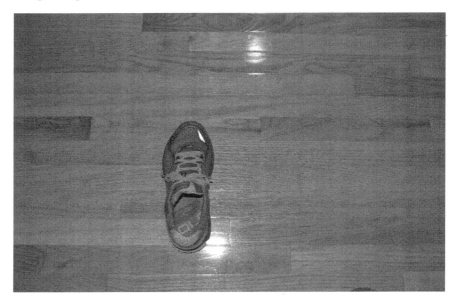

Half kneel

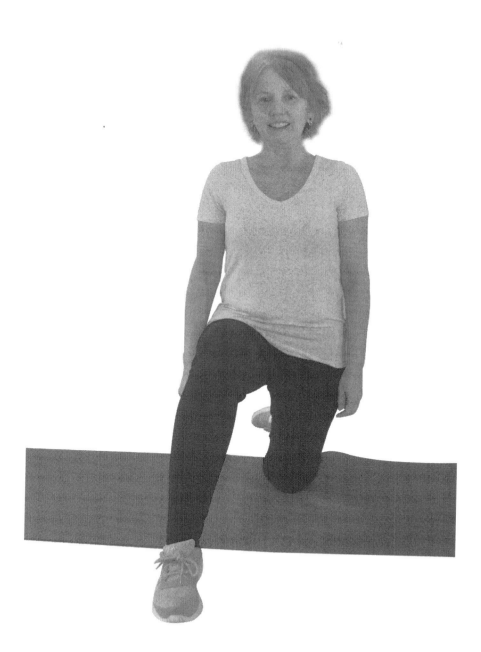

Tall kneel

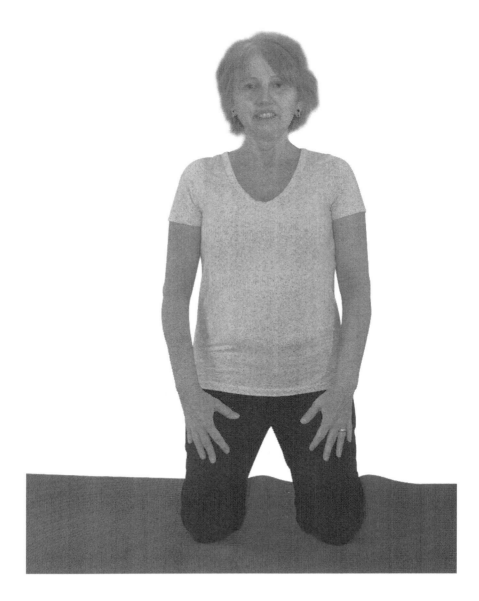

If these positions become too easy, you can increase the challenge by performing these positions with your eyes closed, which improves your balance and proprioception by removing the visual system. Another way to challenge static balance is by adding a secondary task or movement. Do this by turning your head, reaching with your arms, or tapping a balloon while simultaneously maintaining the foot positions.

Our programs incorporate a mix of static and dynamic balance, which allow carryover of strength and balance into your daily life. Our experienced personal trainers will help you determine which aspect of your balance needs the most improvement and challenge you with the appropriate exercises for your needs.

Sample Exercises:

Lunge (with cross body reach)

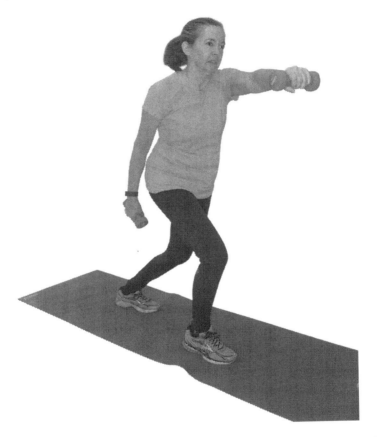

1. Take a large step forward and bend both knees. Do not let your front knee pass your toes. (Beginners can perform a mini lunge as in the picture)
2. Try a few reps before adding a reach across your body.
3. Add light weights for an additional challenge.
4. Do 1-3 sets of 10.

Tandem walk (with head turns)

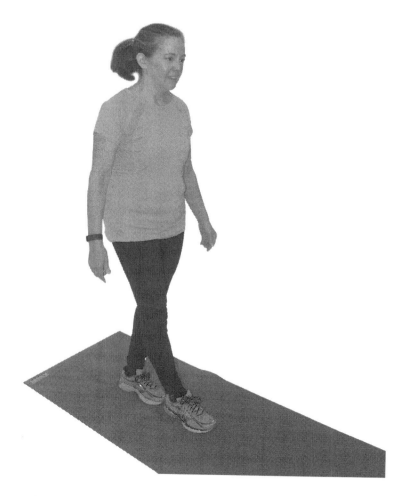

1. Walk forward with heel to toe each step.
2. Try to look ahead.
3. For an added challenge, turn your head side to side as if you are walking in the mall.

Standing cone tap

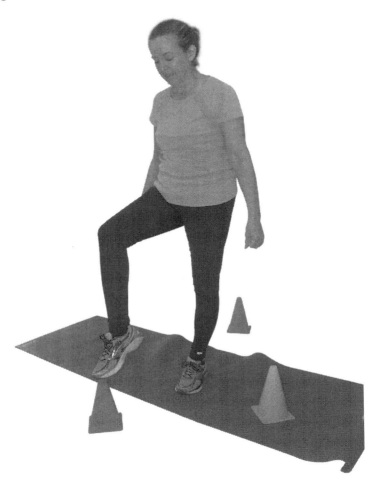

1. Place cones out in 3 points.
2. Stand steady on one foot as you lift the other foot.
3. Gently tap the cone and return your foot to the ground.
4. Then gently tap the next point.
5. For an additional challenge, keep your eyes up and tap all 3 before touching the ground.

Step up (with bicep curl)

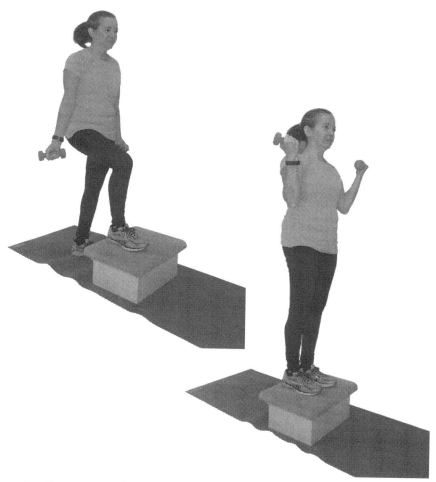

1. Step up with one leg, as you step up perform a bicep curl with light weights.
2. As you step down slowly, lower your arms slowly.
3. Step up quickly and slowly step down 10 times.
4. Do 1-3 sets of 10 reps.

Testimonial:

From her trainer:

When we began working together, Jo Ann wanted to feel her best in the activities she enjoyed before her joint replacement surgeries. Jo Ann had enjoyed hiking and travel. She was very active in her community and church. She felt she could not keep up with her friends in her hiking group and struggled with her balance on the trail. This activity is very challenging because not only did she have to maneuver the different surfaces of the trails, but turn her head simultaneously to take in the sights of nature and obstacles around her. Hiking also requires strength and endurance in her lower body to take these long trips. After working with us, Jo Ann was able to join her family on hiking trips up to the tops of mountains. She also hiked across France with friends!

From Jo Ann:

I started with Vitality after recovering from a knee and a hip replacement. I felt that I needed professional guidance to continue to regain my strength and balance, and to avoid injuring a tender shoulder. My personal trainer provided that guidance and I always felt very confident, as well as challenged, with her instructions.

I am now back to the hiking that I love, and much more mindful that I must "use it or lose it" for the parts of my body that don't do the walking, too.

Jo Ann A.

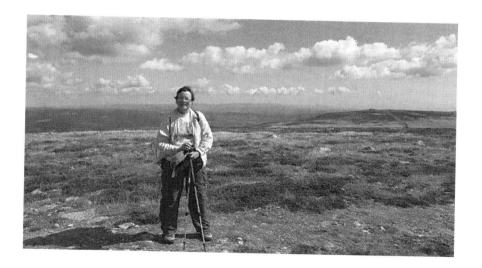

Hiking in France, September 2015

In the photo above, we see Jo Ann thirteen months after knee replacement, eleven months after hip replacement.

"I walked 102 miles on that trip. I thank Vitality Fitness for helping me to regain my strength."

Chapter 4
Strength and Power

"Life is tough, my darling, but so are you."
—Stephanie Bennett Henry

Are stairs becoming more challenging for you? Do you struggle with knee pain? Can you get up and down from the floor with ease? Do you grunt as you get up from the couch? Can you lift the groceries out of the trunk and get them into the house? All of these activities are important parts of our lives. As we age, we lose muscle mass in a process called sarcopenia. Our muscles begin to lose the fibers that regulate strength, power, and endurance. "The typical aging adult will lose around 30 percent of their muscle mass and maximal strength from the time they peak in their thirties to the age of seventy when the decline appears to increase in an accelerated fashion" (Jones 2006).

Research shows that as we age we lose more type II, fast-twitch, muscle fibers compared to type I, slow-twitch, muscle fibers. Type II muscle fibers are associated with bursts of strength and power whereas type I muscle fibers are responsible for endurance. By maintaining a sedentary lifestyle, one could lose up to ten pounds of muscle mass per decade! (Exercise and Aging: Can you walk away from Father Time? Harvard Health Publications, www.health.harvard.edu) Performing the right resistance and weight-bearing strength exercises allows our bodies to counterbalance this loss and increase strength, power, and daily function.

Principles Important to Strength

Our programs not only address the muscle loss associated with aging, they incorporate three important concepts of fitness: specificity, progressive overload, and power.

You might be thinking, "Hey, this is great and all but I've been exercising for years!" Great! I am glad you have been exercising! You are definitely one of the few that can stay self-motivated. However, are you performing the same exercises each time you work out? How often do you change the resistance or weight you are using? Do you always use the same two-pound hand weights?

Progressive overload requires a gradual increase in the volume, intensity, or frequency of exercise to see a change in muscle tone. This does not mean you will develop bodybuilder muscles when increasing the amount of weight you lift. In order to develop tone in your muscles, you must challenge them by varying the resistance, repetitions, or frequency of strength training. Our trainers know how to guide your body safely through this progressive overload. Pushing you too hard or fast could risk injury.

The next concept of strength training is specificity. In order to become better at a particular exercise or motion, you must perform that exercise or motion to improve. Our programs do not include stationary machines that strengthen one muscle at a time, such as those you might see at the gym. Our exercises move your body through dynamic motions in all three planes of motion to mimic the three-dimensional aspect of life.

The last concept of fitness our programs include is power. Power is taking an exercise one step further from strengthening. It requires power to perform movements like getting up from the floor, up from a low chair, or climbing a high step. The definition of power is force multiplied by velocity; therefore, to achieve power training one must perform a strengthening exercise at a quicker speed. However, power training should only be included in an exercise program once a muscle group has adequate strength.

What is Functional Fitness?

Functional fitness is a type of strength and balance training in which exercise movements mimic motions performed in daily life. Do you want to get back to biking, hiking, gardening, or jogging? Do you want to be able to climb the stairs without pain so you can continue to live in your two-story house? Do you want to have the endurance to travel with family and play with your grandkids? There is great carryover from functional fitness exercises to achieving these goals.

When you are out in the world, motion does not occur in only one plane or with one muscle group at a time. Daily movements are dynamic and always changing. Picking up your grandkids or groceries, moving furniture, and lifting potted plants may be activities you engage in. Awkward angles will occur, the ground will not always be smooth, and you may not always be able to maintain the perfect body and alignment. Functional fitness will help you to be strong for these activities. You will be better prepared for the unexpected. Exercises will involve movement in several planes of motion, dynamic movements, and incorporate several muscle groups at a time. You will find yourself getting through your day with ease and doing activities you never thought you could!

"Register your book at VitalityFitnWell.com to access 3 Bonus Training Videos!"

Sample Exercises:

Sit to stand (with overhead reach)

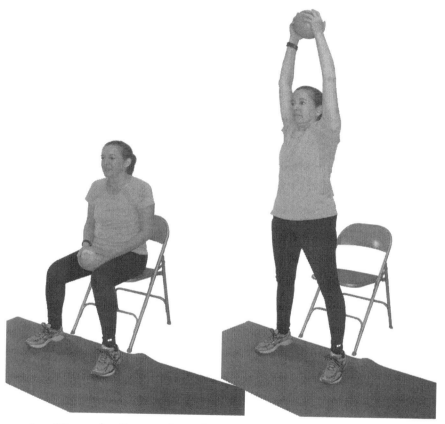

1. Sit on the front edge of a sturdy chair; keep feet shoulder-width apart.
2. Rise to standing position; add overhead lift with ball for a challenge. Can use a weighted ball.
3. Slowly lower to sit.
4. Do 1-3 sets of 10 repetitions.

Wood chops (with medicine ball)

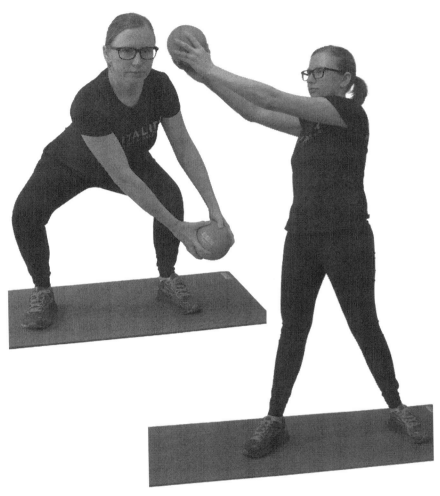

1. Hold ball (weighted for a challenge) in both hands.
2. Squat with hips back; reach down at a diagonal.
3. Rise up squeezing your glutes and raise ball to opposite diagonal. Do not hunch shoulders.
4. Do 1-3 sets of 10. Use weight appropriate for you. Should feel muscles working by 10th rep.

Lunge (with chest press)

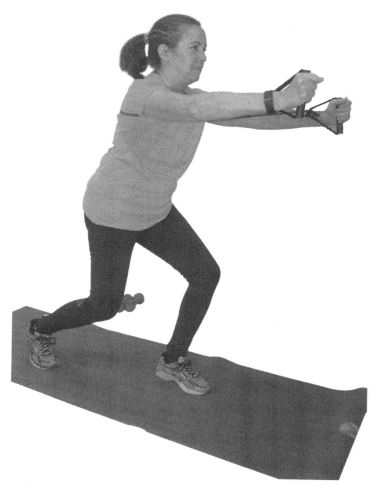

1. Take a large step forward (or a smaller step if starting with mini lunge).
2. Bend knees. Do not let knee go beyond toes.
3. Add chest press with band. Keep elbows up. Press arms forward and slowly let elbows bend upon return.
4. Do 1-3 sets of 10 reps.

Step up (with curl and press)

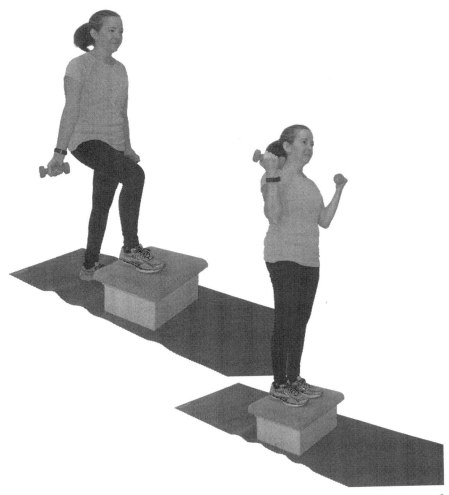

1. Step up with one leg, as you step up perform a bicep curl with light weights.
2. As you step down slowly, lower your arms slowly.
3. Step up quickly and slowly step down 10 times.
4. Do 1-3 sets of 10 reps.

Bridges

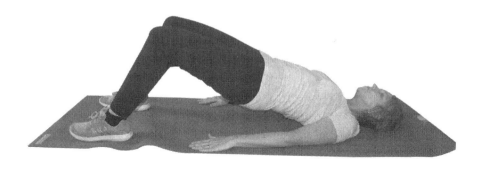

1. Keep feet shoulder-width apart. Tuck stomach muscles in tight. Squeeze glutes.
2. Raise hips and hold 5 seconds.
3. Do 1-3 sets of 10-15.

Unilateral bridges

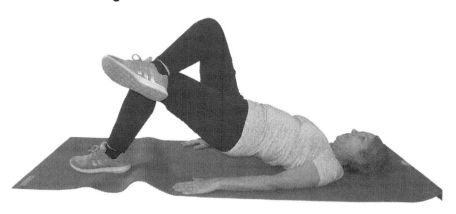

1. Cross one leg over the other. Tuck in stomach muscles and squeeze glutes.
2. Raise hips, keeping them level. Hold for 3 seconds. Do 1-3 sets 10-15 reps.

Bridge with triceps press

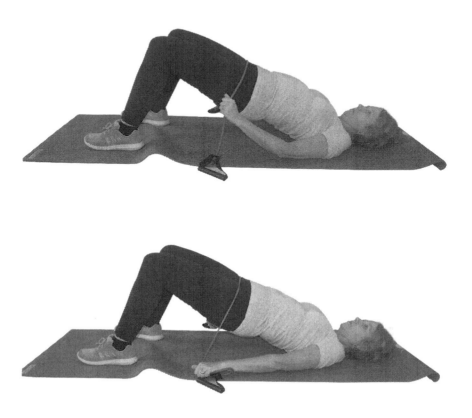

1. Feet shoulder-width apart. Squeeze stomach muscles and glutes.
2. Wrap band over hips. Hold the ends with some resistance. Keep elbows on mat at all times.
3. As you raise your hips, press your arms down slowly. As you lower your hips, slowly return arms to your side.
4. Do 1-3 sets of 10-15 reps.

Chapter 5
What to Expect

"What you do today can improve all your tomorrows."
—THEODORE ROOSEVELT

At this point, you should understand the importance of regular exercise and the types of exercise that are important as we age. It is essential to practice exercises that address posture, balance, and strength. Get started with the great sample exercises in this book. If you do not know where to begin, exercise with a personal trainer who can remove the guesswork and give you quicker results.

What is Small Group Personal Training?

Some people believe that working out with a personal trainer is an exclusive, expensive luxury. However, with small group personal training, sessions with an experienced personal trainer are more affordable for the everyday consumer. Along with the affordability, exercising in a small group provides motivation not only from the trainer, but from a group of your peers as well. Our small groups have three to five participants with one personal trainer.

As in our individual personal training, small group participants will have a one-on-one fitness consultation prior to the sessions in order to review their personal goals and level of fitness. Instead of the cookie-cutter approach seen in many group programs, our personal trainers will guide participants through individualized exercises. Our personal trainers will ensure correct technique and adjust resistance as suited for your fitness level and for your goals. We design your session with your success in view!

Experience by your side!

Have you tried an exercise program in the past and lost your motivation? Has health and fitness been a New Year's resolution time and time again? Has it been years since you have exercised? Eighty percent of people who start a new program at the gym will quit within five months.

Our programs are different from going to the gym because you are not alone! From the group atmosphere to our passionate personal trainers, we offer you the accountability and motivation you need to reach your goals. Our experienced personal trainers are certified Functional Aging Specialists who have the knowledge to safely guide you through the best exercises for your fitness level—this means they are trained to challenge you each session and push you just the right amount to reach your goals. If you are experiencing or recovering from an injury or medical condition, they have the knowledge to choose the proper exercises to help you avoid injury. Our personal trainers are not intimidating because they are passionate about helping you to feel your best.

How do we begin?

When you start with Vitality Fitness, one of our personal trainers will meet with you for an individual consultation. They will review your health history, your goals for fitness and health, and take some measurements of your strength, flexibility, posture, balance, and endurance. We use evidence-based tests with normative data to give you objective information about your current fitness level. Our personal trainers will give you an idea of how long it will take to reach your goals and how often you should be exercising. We have seen the best results with our clients exercising two to three times a week for forty-five minute sessions.

What to expect during my sessions

For your exercise sessions, wear comfortable clothing that allows you to move around easily. A t-shirt and shorts is a good choice. You will move into different positions during your session; double-check yourself for wardrobe malfunctions at home. It is important to wear supportive athletic shoes with a non-slip bottom and, for women, a supportive athletic bra. Bring water and a towel to your sessions, as you will want to stay hydrated and wipe away perspiration. Staying hydrated will also help to reduce muscle aches.

Each small group personal training session is different from your typical big box gym experience. When you come to your session, you will see we do not use exercise machines. We use a variety of equipment including resistance bands, free weights, cones, steps, weighted medicine balls, and your own body weight, which allows you to challenge your muscles through all three planes of movement. Nor do we use typical cardio machines for warm-up as a dynamic movement warm-up is more effective for your cardiovascular system and allows your body to prepare for the exercises in your session.

Sample warm-up:

4-5 minutes, 30 seconds of each

- Standing arm circles, backward
- Trunk rotation, hands clasped
- Big reaches floor to ceiling with mini squats
- Diagonal reaches or wood chops, each side
- Heel kicks
- March in place
- Step tap with alternating arm reaches sideways, overhead
- Small lunge forward
- Small lunge sideways
- Small lunge backward

Good pain vs bad pain

It is important to communicate with your personal trainer when you begin a new exercise program—and throughout. If you are experiencing pain before, during, or after an exercise, your personal trainer needs to know. Our trainers have the experience to modify and adjust exercises or technique as needed. Gone are the days of the "no pain, no gain" mindset.

This theory will only cause injury and frustration leading you to join the statistic of those who tried a new exercise routine and failed.

Listen to your body for signals. There is a difference between "good pain" and "bad pain." "Good pain" is the soreness or "burn" you feel in your muscle belly when you are performing an exercise. One to two days after a good workout, you may feel muscle belly soreness that resolves within a day or two. Delayed onset muscle soreness or DOMS is not a cause for concern and is a normal part of a good exercise routine. This is a signal that your muscles are remodeling and becoming stronger.

On the other hand, "bad pain" occurs in your joints, not the muscle belly, and is a more severe pain. If you experience "bad pain" with an exercise, your body is signaling you to stop right away. Keep open communication with your personal trainer; often they can guide you through a change in position to avoid this pain. If you continue to experience "bad pain," it is best to check in with your doctor, as it could be a sign of something more serious.

Safety, red flags:

When beginning a new exercise program, safety is the most important consideration. Be sure to check with your doctor before beginning any exercise program.

Please stop your workout, let your trainer know, and contact your doctor if you feel any of these symptoms before, during, or after a workout:

- Dizziness
- Nausea/Vomiting

- Chest pain or tightness
- Unusual shortness of breath
- Pain in neck or jaw or radiating down the left arm

Chapter 6
Why Our Approach is Different

"It is health that is the real wealth,
and not pieces of gold and silver."
—MAHATMA GANDHI

From your appearance, to your health and safety, to the energy and endurance your body needs, exercise is important as we age. The most important reason is enabling your body to stay strong to enjoy activities you are passionate about for many years to come. Whether your passion is travel, gardening, hiking, family time, or golf and tennis, the benefits of exercise will allow you to enjoy these activities so much more! Reinvent aging with us. Lose those aches and pains, improve your balance, and get the energy you need to keep up with your friends, family and loved ones every day.

Peace of mind

You can find excellent personal trainers, but you may also find trainers with little to no experience who could put you at risk for injury. We need national regulation for personal trainers. How frustrating would it be to make the decision to begin an exercise program, hire a personal trainer, and end up with an injury that you have to rehab for a year or more? Our experienced personal trainers provide a safe option for older adults, where you can feel confident and trust the guidance of your personal trainer.

Our personal trainers hold the highest certifications as certified personal trainers. They are also Functional Aging Specialists. Functional Aging Specialist is an in-depth, evidence-based certification that focuses on the needs of older adults. We understand that your priorities in health and fitness may be different from those of someone in their twenties, but the days of sitting in a chair with one-pound dumbbells for 'senior fitness' are gone. We guide our clients through exercises starting with basic concepts of movement to ensure correct technique and progressing to more complex movements and combinations of exercises. Our personal trainers have the knowledge to guide you through the right exercises for your needs.

You will not only feel safe with our personal trainers, they will keep you accountable to your goals. Has your doctor recommended exercise? Do you have a health condition that could benefit from regular exercise? We all know the benefits of exercise, so why aren't we doing it? It is not easy to stay motivated in a world with so many distractions. Having a personal trainer keeps you accountable with a regular schedule for exercise and provides the motivation you need to reach your goals.

Do you find the gym intimidating? The loud music, the confusing machines, and the crowd can be daunting. Our programs work in small peer groups. Many of our clients have similar goals and there are shared core components of exercise that everyone needs, but we understand that a cookie-cutter approach will not work. Each person has specific goals and desires for their life, and is starting at their own fitness level. We customize sessions to match your needs and push you just the right amount.

Improve your "do-ability!"

Our programs will help tone your body, improve your balance, decrease your risk of injury, reduce aches and pains, and give you the confidence to live life to the fullest. We want to help you Reinvent Aging.

"Register your book at VitalityFitnWell.com to access 3 Bonus Training Videos!"

Chapter 7
Testimonials

I am in a new relationship with someone older than me and I realized that he has more energy than me! I want to keep up with him. Also, I want to look my best at my son's wedding this summer! I am enjoying the work out in small groups and my trainer is great! At first, I thought that since I wasn't sweating much, I wasn't getting that much of a work out. But, then, the next morning I am so sore! I'm using all these muscles that I didn't know I had! Thanks so much!

N.L.

My training sessions are great! My trainer in the groups knows just how much to push me. He is attentive to technique and I feel my muscles working. He has just the right way of motivating you.

L.S.

I had a great time at my training sessions with a small group! It was so fun, it didn't feel like a workout but later I could feel all the benefits!

R.W.

I am really thrilled with small group personal training and find my trainer to be an expert in explaining things. He's so friendly and encouraging. I find its at the right level for me and my trainer is very in tune with what he thinks I can and cannot do. I was leery of having a "cookie cutter" style trainer who would not take into account my personal inabilities.

E.C.

I have had issues with my back and symptoms down my leg. After physical therapy, I joined the small group personal training with Vitality Fitness. I can say that my right leg is getting stronger and there is less intense pain and inflammation in the thigh and right hip since I started with the groups. The majority of time I can climb the stairs and not feel a weakness in the right thigh and leg. My doctor and I agreed I wouldn't take another round of steroids since I'm seeing progress from my exercise. I believe my sessions are extremely beneficial for me.

K.L.

I started going to Vitality Fitness for my back. I found that I was unable to take moderate to long walks without pain. In fact I could not even walk past the neighbors house without my back starting to hurt and would turn around and go back into my house. Last week my wife and I went on a trip and did a lot of walking and my back never bothered me once. In fact, when I checked my phone for the number of steps that I took I had taken more than 7000 steps a day. My trainer has done a great job with me and I really appreciate all of her efforts to help me. I would strongly recommend Vitality Fitness to any older adult with back problems.

T.A.

Vitality Fitness has helped me with balance and confidence. I have not fallen since starting the program and previously I was having falls periodically. Also important is the confidence I now have in walking. I no longer use my cane outside. When I step on uneven places on the sidewalk I am able to recover quickly without falling. Love the sessions and my personal trainer with Vitality Fitness.

G.E.

I came to Vitality because I took one of their balance classes. It was very informative and well run. I wanted to take more balance classes and I liked the concept that Vitality specialized in exercising older adults in small groups. After my in depth, one-on-one fitness consultation with my personal trainer, I then had to decide if I should take classes with Vitality or the exercise person which was recommended by my physical therapist. I really liked Vitality's philosophies on what older adults CAN do and how we need to break down exercises and perform them in steps, in order to continue doing the things we love (dancing, tennis, biking, hiking or soccer with the Grandkids) safely. Doctors sometimes limit us by restricting our movements to "keep us safe." Needless to say, I went with Vitality. My trainer has been a wonderful teacher and she has given me good advice on many issues dealing with health and wellness. I trust her to push me just the right amount depending on the day. She makes exercising fun and purposeful. Her attention to detail, her thoughtful advice, her sincere caring, her smile, laugh and dedication all contribute to motivating me. I now exercise every morning (I do about twenty minutes of balance exercises) in addition to my two Vitality sessions, a weekly yoga class and a weekly aerobics class.

E.F.

Reinvent Aging

21 Days to Improve Your Energy, Strength, and Balance!

If you are ready to finally wake up without stiffness, pain-free, and full of energy, don't miss our next **21 Day Transformation Challenge.**

As a valued reader of my book, take action and grab your VIP pass today to enjoy a 21-day body tune-up at 40% off!

Your journey includes:

✓ Health Assessment
✓ Goal Setting
✓ Nutrition Support and Meal Plan
✓ Expert Exercise Guidance

Visit VitalityVIP.com to Apply or Call 240-293-0982

Two Convenient Locations in Montgomery County!

Limited Space Available, Apply Today!

About the Author

Aubrey is a certified personal trainer through NCCPT, a licensed Physical Therapist Assistant, a certified Senior Fitness Specialist through NASM, and a Functional Aging Specialist through the Functional Aging Institute. She received her bachelor's degree from Moravian College. While working as a Physical Therapist Assistant, Aubrey founded Vitality Fitness and Wellness to respond to the need for year-round wellness for healthy adults along with those who were recovering from medical conditions. She is certified in LSVT Big treatment for individuals with Parkinson's Disease. She is a mom of two young children, Skyler and Colbie, her dachshund, Leonard, and cat, Chloe. She is passionate about her work with older adults and brings an enthusiasm to encourage you to be committed to stay active for life!

Vitality Fitness offers one-on-one and small group personal training as well as balance classes. Give us a call today! 240-293-0982 VitalityFitnWell.com

68320120R00048

Made in the USA
Lexington, KY
10 October 2017